How A Honey Bun Almost Took Me Out

The Humorous yet real story of being diagnosed and living with type 2 diabetes

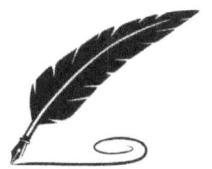

RENEA L. MOSS

Attitude Publishing

A DIVISION OF MIXED BAG ENTERPRISES

© 2025 Renea L. Moss

All rights reserved.

No part of this publication may be reproduced, distributed, or transmitted in any form or by any means—electronic, mechanical, photocopying, recording, or otherwise—without the prior written permission of the author, except in the case of brief quotations used in critical articles or reviews.

Publisher:: Attitude Publishing

ISBN: 978-0-9849502-3-2

Printed in the United States of America

This book is written as a source of information only. The information contained in this book should by no means be considered a substitute for the advice of a qualified medical professional, who should always be consulted before beginning any new diet, exercise, or other health program.

All efforts have been made to ensure the accuracy of the information contained in this book as of the date of publication. The author and the publisher expressly disclaim responsibility for any adverse effects arising from the use or application of the information contained herein.

For inquiries, appearances, or bulk purchases, contact:

✉ renea.moss@reneasworld.com

⊕ www.reneasworld.com | @RaiRenea

DEDICATION

To the women who've cried over fries, made shady deals with rice, and silently judged a honey bun like it was their ex—

For the warrior women who carry glucose tabs in one pocket and hope in the other.

To the woman who counts carbs like blessings, stares at labels like fortune tellers, and still finds time to dance

To every woman balancing life, blood sugar, and everybody else's needs—may this book be your mirror, your laugh, and your light. this is your redemption story!

FOREWORD

Before I could ever write about the Honey Bun that almost took me out…

Before I could crack a joke about ashy skin, sugar spikes, or saying goodbye to Wingstop…

I had to write this.

Because beneath the laughs, the side-eyes, and the sass, there is always truth. There is always that whisper inside asking:

Can I really do this?

Can I carry this diagnosis, this fear, this change?

Can I survive it—and still be me?

So, before we dive into all the glucose, grit, and glory, I wanted to start with this poem.

It's not a cute Instagram caption.

It's not a motivational quote for your bathroom mirror.

It's the truth. My truth.

When I was first diagnosed with Type 2 Diabetes, I didn't feel strong or brave. I felt like a fraud with a honey bun in my purse and shame in my chest. I wasn't ready to be the "hero" of my own story—I was just trying to stay conscious.

This poem was written in one of those moments.

When I felt exposed. Unworthy.

When I realized the version of me people cheered for wasn't always the same one crying in the bathroom or Googling "can you go into a coma from eating one cupcake?"

But I shared it anyway—because somebody out there is wearing the same smile while hiding the same fear.

So if you read this and feel seen, scared, or even slightly empowered…

Know that you don't have to be perfect to be powerful.

And surviving—even when it's messy—is still a miracle.

And so, I offer you this poem—raw, reflective, and real—as the heart behind the humor.

This isn't just the Foreword to a book.

It's a foreword to vulnerability. To resilience.

To not knowing all the answers—but showing up anyway.

HERO

"There's a hero", the songwriter tells me. "If you look inside your heart you don't have to be afraid of what you are!" That a hero will come along and give me the strength to carry; if I cast my fears aside then I'll know that I can…….

Survive???

Well, I really just don't know

Even though you see

A picture of self-confidence written all over me

It's just not true

I am quivering inside

Wondering if I can live up

To the person I know I can be

Not afraid that I may disappoint you

But more afraid that I may disappoint me!

I hear the talk all around me

Of the inner spirit

And yeah, it sounds good

But can I live up to the reality

Of this Goddess

That everyone else has projected on me

In one instance I want to grow

And project that inner beauty

But all the while I'm having urges of

Backing that 'ass up' on the scene

Wondering if it's just lies I'm feeding the audience

Let alone to me!

Pondering my self-realization

Asking myself can I live up to my poetry

Or is my poetry too deep

Even for me

So I look inside my heart for that hero

And I am afraid that I will find a villain

And with that fear, I will never get the answers

Because I am afraid that I won't find anything

Not even a soul

Just an illusion of what others think I should be

Without ever really finding me!

Thus, I continue

To hide my self-doubt and sorrow

With a smile

Making you believe that everything is O.K.

All the while knowing

I'm just trying to survive for the day

Thus, I come before you

Standing here

Weaving stories and tales

For you to hear

Inspiring you to succeed

With pen and paper

My insecurities disappear

And I erase my inner need

Making you feel good about yourself

If only for the moment

Making you envy me

For my use of similes

Making you think

I am in control of my destiny

Because my metaphoric verbiage

gives me a greater than life image to see!

But all the while

I am hoping

That you will be my hero

That you will look past

The smile and terminology

And know

THAT I AM SCARED

That I could never live up

to the words in my poetry

I want you to know that my poetry

Doesn't define me!

I just use everyday words

To discuss

the dreams

the thoughts

and inner demons

inside all of us!

As I stand here

Being your hero

Giving credence

to the inner fears

That you won't let go

Helping you escape the demons

That is haunting your cerebral being

Inspiring you to move past those things

That stops you from reaching

The potential of your being

With pen and paper in hand

I'm your hero in poetry land

Using my supernatural powers to weave and deceive

And make you believe

What I want you to believe

But when I walk off that stage

Put my glasses on

And become

Ms. Claire Kent

I want you to know

That I am waiting

On my Superman

My Hero

To come and save me

From my predicament!

SURVIVE??

I just don't know

Because the Goddess

That you see before you

Is trembling inside

Hoping

And

Praying

THAT

SHE

can fulfill

HER DESTINY!

And now, as you turn the page into my story—may it meet you where you are, speak to what you may not have said out loud, and remind you:

You're not alone.

We're walking this out together.

Ashy ankles, glucose monitors, and all.

Welcome to my story.

Welcome to The Honey Bun Redemption.

Renea L. Moss

Table of Contents

Dedication -- 3

Foreword -- 4

Chapter 1: The Honey Bun That Tried To Kill Me ---------- 15

Chapter 2: The Great Pee Emergency ------------------------ 19

Chapter 3: The Thirst Is Real ---------------------------------- 23

Chapter 4: Ashy Ain't Cute ------------------------------------- 27

Chapter 5: Itching Where The Sun Don't Shine ------------ 33

Chapter 6: Blink Twice If You Can See Me -------------------- 39

Chapter 7: Puff, Puff… Nope – The Swelling Nobody Talks About --- 45

Chapter 8: When Fine Met Phema --------------------------- 51

Chapter 8 (Deeper Cut): The Weight Drop That Made Me Cute Then Insulin Said "Psych" – Ft. Ozempic Lies & Real-Life Results --- 57

Chapter 9: Double Trouble – When Diabetes Brings Along High Blood Pressure -- 61

Chapter 10: The Wingstop Breakup --------------------------- 67

Chapter 11: Pills, Prayers And Process Of Elimination --- 75

Chapter 12: "I Don't Look Sick" – Fighting A Disease That People Can't See --- 81

Chapter 13: Diabetic Guilt, Shame, And The "Should've Known Better" Spiral --- 87

Chapter 14: Sex, Skin & Sugar – The Intimate Side Of Diabetes -- *91*

Chapter 15: Love, Lust, And The Low Sugar Text – Dating & Relationships With Diabetes -------------------------- *97*

Chapter 16: The Diabetes Survival Kit – What's In Your Bag, Sis? --- *101*

Chapter 17: The 7 Types Of Diabetic Days – A Humorous Breakdown --- *105*

Final Chapter: Still Sweet – A Message From Me To You --- *111*

Chapter 1

The Honey Bun That Tried to Kill Me

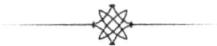

I was just trying to live my best life. One last honey bun, I told myself. Just one. But no—my body said, "Girl, if you don't sit down somewhere…" Next thing I knew, the world tilted, and my blood sugar was doing backflips. A tale of rebellion, regret, and almost passing out.

More than **1 in 10 Americans** have diabetes—but I didn't know I was one of them until a honey bun nearly took me out like a bad ex. I had just gotten the diagnosis. Did I listen to the doctor? Well, yes and no. I was good for two weeks after being released from the hospital. Then, one day, as I was walking past a vending machine, I locked eyes with that sticky, glazed piece of temptation and whispered, "One more won't kill me." Turns out, it almost did. I almost blacked out with half a honey bun in my mouth and a sugar level so high it could've powered a Tesla. That's when I knew this wasn't a game. Diabetes had entered the chat—and it brought receipts.

The Setup

Let me back up. The day I was diagnosed, I didn't cry. I didn't get scared. I got *mad*. Mad because I felt fine. Mad because nobody warned me about this. Mad because—let's be real—how many of us grew up with plates full of starch, sugar, and "don't waste no food"? Diabetes felt like a betrayal. And I wasn't ready to give up my favorite snacks just yet. Especially not my honey buns. Those soft, gooey, microwave-for-10-seconds, "I'm just gonna have one" honey buns.

So I rebelled. Bought one, sat by the pool, and took a bite like I was in a music video. Halfway through, my head got light. My heart was beating funny. I was sweating, and not in a cute way. I thought maybe it was stress or the heat. But when I started seeing black spots and felt like I was floating, I knew something was wrong.

The Crash

What was I feeling? That was a blood sugar spike—*and* crash. A lot of people think diabetes just means your sugar is high, but it's not that simple. Your blood sugar jumps up after you eat, especially when it's straight sugar and processed carbs like, well… a honey bun. And if your body can't produce or properly use insulin, it can't get that sugar into your cells for energy. So, instead of feeding your body, the sugar stays in your bloodstream and wreaks havoc.

That "floaty" feeling? That was my body waving a red flag. *Sis, we are not okay.*

The Aftermath

I somehow made it to my bedroom, laid on the bed, and didn't move for hours. My head was pounding. I felt weak, dizzy, and low-key scared. I had visions of my tombstone that read, "A Honoeybun took her out." That night, I didn't eat dinner. I didn't touch another honey bun. I just sat with the realization that I wasn't invincible. My body was changing. And if I didn't change with it, I wasn't going to make it.

The Wake-Up Call

What hit me the hardest wasn't the near-pass-out. It was the realization that I had *no idea* how food worked anymore. Nobody sat me down and said, "Here's what you can eat now." I got a diagnosis and a printout. That's it. So I did what most of us do—I Googled. I cried. I tried to find food that didn't taste like cardboard. I messed up. And I kept going.

Mini Pep Talk:

If you've ever tried to sneak a snack and ended up regretting it, you're not alone. This journey comes with cravings, mistakes, and moments that humble you real quick. But it also comes with chances to do better, to *feel* better, and to take control—even if it's one bite at a time.

✅ Quick Checklist: Signs Your Blood Sugar Might Be Too High

1. 😵 Dizziness or lightheadedness after eating
2. Sweating for no clear reason
3. 💤 Feeling sleepy after snacks
4. Craving sugar even when you just ate
5. 🚨 Feeling "off" after high-carb meals

💬 Real Talk Reflection Prompt

Have you ever eaten something you knew you shouldn't... and immediately regretted it? Write that moment down. What did you learn from it?

📣 Pull Quote

"I blacked out with half a honey bun in my mouth and a sugar level so high it could've powered a Tesla."

Chapter 2

The Great Pee Emergency

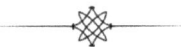

Frequent urination like never before—when you can't make it to the bathroom and start planning your life around pee breaks. I used to laugh at those commercials where people "can't hold it." Now I *am* the commercial. If there's a bathroom within a mile radius, I know about it. If not, I'm in danger.

They don't tell you that diabetes means planning your life around bathrooms. They don't tell you that you'll know where every clean toilet is in a five-mile radius like it's a personal superpower. And they *definitely* don't tell you that you'll have moments where you're standing in a parking lot, doing the Pee-Pee Two-Step, trying to decide between public embarrassment or sprinting like your bladder depends on it—because it does.

I went from casually sipping water like a dainty queen to running to the bathroom every 15 minutes like it was cardio. And no, I wasn't pregnant. I was diabetic and in denial. I thought I just had a small bladder or a messed up kidney.. *Spoiler alert*: It was high blood sugar, not hydration.

The Day I Peed Myself (Yes, We're Going There)

Let me set the scene: grocery store, long line, just two items in my hand—some unsweetened almond milk and a cucumber (don't judge me). I *felt* the pressure building, but I figured I could make it through the line.

Wrong.

Out of nowhere, my body said, "Release the flood." And baby, it did. Right there between Aisle 3 and Checkout Lane 2, I peed my damn pants. Not a cute little drip. A full-on, shame-filled, middle-school-nightmare-style *whoosh*. I dropped the almond milk and ran out like the building was on fire.

At the time, I didn't know my blood sugar was through the roof, and my kidneys were working overtime trying to flush it out. That's what diabetes does—it makes your body try to pee out the sugar it can't process. It's called **polyuria**, and it's one of the first signs of diabetes. And guess what? **Black Americans are more likely to experience complications from uncontrolled diabetes**, partly because our symptoms are misdiagnosed or flat-out ignored.

The Science-y Part (But Still Real)

When your blood sugar is high, your body tries to push the extra sugar out through your urine. That means you're peeing. A lot. And with all that peeing comes dehydration. So guess what? You get thirsty. Which means you drink more water. And then you pee more. Congratulations, you're now in the *Bathroom Olympics*, and there is no gold medal.

I was in the restroom so much that I started naming the stalls. "Oh hey, Stall #2, long time no see."

When It Gets Real

There's nothing cute about not being able to control your bladder. There's nothing fun about waking up four times a night, stumbling to the bathroom, and bumping into walls like a drunk toddler. And there's absolutely nothing funny about peeing yourself—but I laugh now because I *have* to.

That moment in the grocery store humbled me. It also sent me back to the doctor, who looked at my glucose levels and said, "Ma'am... your sugar is *how* high?" I left with a new prescription, a plan, and the sudden desire to never be more than five feet from a restroom.

Let's Be Honest...

We don't talk about this stuff enough—especially as Black women. We're taught to "hold it," to power through, to be strong and silent. But ignoring symptoms like this can lead to real damage, like kidney problems or even nerve issues. Peeing all the time isn't just annoying—it's your body trying to save itself.

Mini Pep Talk:

If you're peeing like your bladder is on a time clock, you're not nasty, weak, or broken. You're just dealing with something real. And the good news? With the right meds, food, and support, that *gotta-go* urgency *can* calm down. Trust me—I'm finally reclaiming my right to grocery shop without fear of a bladder rebellion.

✅ Bathroom Survival Tips

1. 🚻 Know where public bathrooms are before leaving home
2. 🧻 Pack extra undies or liners—just in case
3. ⚫ Balance hydration without overloading sugar (watch the juices!)
4. 📱 Track your blood sugar spikes after meals

Did You Know?

The average adult urinates 4–7 times a day. If you're going 10+ times, especially at night, it may be a sign of high blood sugar.

💬 Real Talk Reflection Prompt

Where were you when you first realized your pee game had changed? What did it feel like physically and emotionally?

📣 Pull Quote

"I started naming the stalls. 'Oh hey, Stall #2, long time no see.'"

Yesss, let's roll right into it—this one's about the thirst that no amount of water seems to fix. And no, we're not talking about Instagram thirst traps. We're talking about the "I just drank 3 bottles of water, and I'm still parched like I ate a fistful of cinnamon" kind of thirst.

Chapter 3

The Thirst Is Real

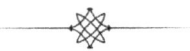

Drinking water like you just crossed a desert... and still feeling like a sponge in the Sahara. I wasn't just thirsty—I was *parched*. Dry mouth, dry soul, dry life. I could drink an ocean and still feel like I needed a sip of something cold. And don't get me started on waking up in the middle of the night for water *and* a bathroom trip.

I was drinking water like it was going out of style. Gallons. Bottles. I was that girl with the emotional-support water jug the size of a toddler. And still, I felt like I'd been crawling through the desert every 10 minutes.

At first, I thought maybe I was just being "healthy." You know, #HydrationGoals. Then I realized something was off when I was drinking more water than Beyoncé's backup dancers and STILL felt like my tongue was made of cotton balls.

The Never-Ending Cycle

Drink water. Run to the bathroom. Drink more water. Run again. I was stuck in this exhausting loop that felt like punishment. And the worst part? *I was still thirsty*. Like mouth-dry, lips-crusty, throat-screaming thirsty.

It wasn't until my doctor said, "Your blood sugar is basically syrup," that I understood what was happening. My body wasn't hydrating—it was fighting.

Why Diabetes Makes You So Thirsty

This symptom has a name: **polydipsia**. Basically, when your blood sugar is high, your body tries to dilute the sugar in your bloodstream by pulling water from your cells. It's like your body's personal fire department trying to put out a sugar fire with every drop of water it can find.

That's why you feel dry and dehydrated no matter how much you drink. And because your kidneys are trying to flush out the sugar too, you end up peeing more—*and* losing more water. That's how diabetes traps you in the great "Pee & Sip" cycle of doom.

Dehydrated and Ashy? Double Whammy

Not only was I drinking like a cactus in crisis, but my skin started to betray me too. Dry. Itchy. Flaky. Ashy like I hadn't seen lotion since the 90s. I started carrying lotion in every bag, car, and room. My elbows looked like they'd been sanding drywall.

It all clicked when I realized this was part of the same problem—when your body is constantly trying to flush sugar, it's drying *everything* out. Your mouth, your skin, even your eyeballs.

A Quick Note for Black Folks

Let's be real: we're used to dry skin being "normal." We joke about being ashy, but for people with diabetes—especially Black people—it's a sign. The thirst, the dryness, the constant need for water and lotion? That's not just winter. That's not just "forgot to moisturize." That might be your blood sugar talking.

How I Got My Life (and Hydration) Together

Once I realized the thirst wasn't just thirst, I started checking my blood sugar every time I felt it hit. And sure enough, it was always high when I was the most parched.

I started switching from juices and flavored drinks to plain water with lemon. I added low-glycemic fruits to help with hydration. And I asked my doctor for a proper blood sugar management plan. Within weeks, I could drink water and actually feel hydrated again. My lips stopped cracking. My skin stopped flaking. And I finally got some peace.

Mini Pep Talk:

If you're drinking like a fish but still feeling dry, you're not crazy—you're *probably* glucose-saturated. Listen to your body. That thirst is a signal, not a flaw. You deserve to feel hydrated, healthy, and like your lips don't need a layer of Vaseline thick enough to stop a windstorm.

✅ Hydration Hacks

Did You Know?

Dehydration can actually raise your blood sugar—and high blood sugar causes more dehydration. Break the cycle with balanced fluid intake.

💬 Real Talk Reflection Prompt

How does thirst show up in your body? How do you know when it's more than "just need a sip"?

📣 Pull Quote

"I was drinking like a cactus in crisis, and still felt like my tongue was made of cotton balls."

Let's gooo! Time to talk about one of the sneakiest, most **disrespectful** *symptoms of them all...*

Chapter 4

Ashy Ain't Cute

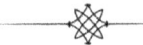

Dry, flaky, itchy skin that makes you question if you even bathed today (you did... twice).

You ever look down at your leg and think, "Did I bathe today?" Not because you actually forgot—but because your skin looks like you've been kicking flour.

Pre-Diagnosis Chronicles: The Ashy Educator Era

Before I knew anything about blood sugar or kidneys or glucose monitors, I was just walking around... flaky. I'm talking *ashy*. Elbow dust, ankle chalk, white-knuckle winter—even in summer.

Now, let me paint this picture: I work with students. High schoolers. Which means if you're ashy, someone will tell you. Out loud. With no mercy.

I became known as the "ashy teacher." Then, the "ashy principal." And yes—I carried lotion everywhere. Purse, desk drawer, glove compartment, emergency bottle under my desk. If there was a layer of skin showing, it was getting moisturized... eventually.

But my students? Oh, they had jokes.

One day, one of my boldest babies looked me dead in the eye and said:

"Ms. Moss, do you even got a man? 'Cause if you do, he not doing his job. He's supposed to be lotioning your feet."

I laughed. Loud. But the truth is—I was moisturizing constantly and *still* dry. I didn't realize that the high blood sugar was dehydrating me from the inside out. That "ashy" wasn't just me forgetting shea butter—it was my body begging for help.

Looking back, it was one of my earliest signs. Before the Pee-Pee Two-Step, before the almond milk incident in Aisle 3… I was dry. As hell. And no amount of lotion could fix what my pancreas was doing.

That was me. I was dry in places I didn't know could get dry. I'm talkin' *ashy elbows, scaly shins, itchy back, flaky shoulders,* and let's not even talk about the heels. I could've started a side hustle as a human chalkboard.

At first, I thought maybe I needed to exfoliate more. Drink more water. Change my soap. But after the tenth day of rubbing on lotion and still feeling like I was shedding like a snake? I knew something deeper was going on.

When Ashiness Becomes a Medical Symptom

The dryness wasn't just cosmetic—it was my skin begging for help. Turns out, high blood sugar doesn't just mess with your internal organs. It messes with your largest organ: **your skin**.

Diabetes can reduce circulation, especially to the hands and feet. Less circulation means less moisture. Plus, your body is working overtime to flush out excess sugar, so it's drying you out from the inside. Add a few sugar spikes and poof! You're a walking bag of desert dust.

The Scratch That Won't Quit

It wasn't just dry—it was *itchy*. I scratched my legs so much I started looking like I fought a cactus and lost. And of course, being a Black woman, I couldn't even hide it. The ash glowed in the light. I felt like I had to lotion in layers just to make it out the house.

I even had that one emergency moment in public—started scratching my ankle through my jeans like a raccoon with a grudge. I knew then: something had to give.

Skin SOS: Why It Happens

1. ● **Dehydration** from frequent urination = dry skin.
2. **Poor circulation** = less natural oil distribution.
3. **Increased risk of skin infections** = extra irritation.
4. **High blood sugar** affects collagen production and skin's healing process.

And guess what? **Black skin is more prone to visible dryness**—but the medical world often doesn't take our complaints seriously. We get handed cocoa butter and vibes instead of actual care plans.

How I Got My Glow Back

- Switched to fragrance-free soap and thick cream (hello shea butter + ceramides)

- Drank water *consistently* (not just during the thirst attacks)

- Started checking my sugar when my skin flared up—it was always high

- Used a humidifier at night (a game-changer in winter)

- Saw a dermatologist who *understood melanin*

Once my sugar started stabilizing, I noticed the itching backed off. The ash? Still shows up if I slack on lotion, but it's no longer a sign of my body screaming from the inside out.

Mini Pep Talk:

If you feel like your skin is betraying you, you're not alone. Dry, itchy skin isn't just a "Black people problem" or a "winter thing." It's a diabetes thing. And it's fixable. You deserve to feel soft, soothed, and NOT like a lizard in shedding season.

🔧 Interactive Elements

✅ Glow-Up Skin Checklist

1. ☐ Thick, fragrance-free lotion (look for "for diabetic skin")
2. 🚿 Skip hot showers—they strip moisture
3. 🌬 Use a humidifier, especially at night
4. 💧 Track hydration with water goals
5. Check blood sugar when itching increases

🎁 Ashy Emergency Kit

- Travel-size lotion or body butter
- Hydrating face mist
- Shea butter stick (for knuckles & elbows!)
- Scratch-safe cotton gloves or socks for sleep

💬 Real Talk Reflection Prompt

When was the last time you felt truly good in your skin—literally and emotionally? What might get you closer to that feeling again?

Did You Know?

Up to **33% of people with diabetes** experience skin-related symptoms before even being diagnosed.

☐ Pull Quote

"I didn't need a shower—I needed insulin."

Alright—let's dive headfirst (but gently 😊) into the realest, most under-discussed symptom of them all...

Chapter 5

Itching Where the Sun Don't Shine

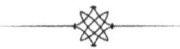

Let's talk about *that* itch. The one you can't explain, but you *feel* in your soul (and your underwear). You ever scratch so hard you start seeing stars? I'm talking about an itch that makes you reevaluate your entire existence. And the worst part? You can't even talk about it without people making *that* face.

Let's just say it: nobody told me that diabetes would have me wanting to scratch my lady parts like I was auditioning for a Monistat commercial.

I'm talkin' full-on, can't-sit-still, ready-to-grab-a-hairbrush itchy. You know that "this must be demonic warfare" kind of itch? That was me. I was trying every trick—coconut oil, powder, sitting with a fan between my legs like I was cooling a pie on a windowsill. Nothing helped. I didn't want to say anything because, well… how do you bring that up in conversation?

"Hi, I have diabetes and my coochie feels like it's allergic to air."

The Quiet Symptom with a Loud Voice

Here's the truth: high blood sugar makes you a buffet for yeast. And guess what yeast loves? Warm, moist places. Vaginas are already a 5-star hotel for yeast if the balance is off. Add uncontrolled glucose to the mix, and baby—it's an overbooked resort.

And yet… nobody warned me. Nobody at the doctor's office said, "By the way, you might feel like you want to rub your whole crotch off with a loofah." I had to find out the hard way—through trial, error, and Google searches like *"why does my coochie hate me?"*

The Stats Behind the Itch

Here's where it gets real:

- **Up to 75% of women** with diabetes experience recurring **yeast infections** or **vaginal thrush**.
- **Black women are more likely to go undiagnosed** or misdiagnosed when reporting vaginal discomfort—too often written off as "hygiene" issues rather than real metabolic symptoms.

The over-the-counter creams might give you temporary relief, but until you address your **blood sugar**, the yeast will keep coming back like it paid rent.

The Embarrassment Factor

I know how hard it is to talk about this. It's not cute. It's not "Instagram awareness post" material. But it's real. And if I felt like I was the only one? I *know* some of y'all out there are silently suffering too. That itching, burning, uncomfortable "why-me" feeling doesn't make you dirty—it makes you human. A human with diabetes and a vagina that deserves respect.

And let's be clear: this ain't just about vaginas. Men with diabetes get jock itch and dry, irritated skin in their private areas too. Nobody's exempt.

Itching. Burning. Dryness. Discomfort.

And not in a sexy, Fifty Shades of Grey kind of way.

Sometimes it felt like my body was mad at me. I was doing "all the things"—taking my meds, drinking my water—and still dealing with:

- Yeast infections on repeat like a toxic ex
- That unbearable itchy feeling that makes you want to rub yourself raw
- White discharge that had me Googling everything at 3 a.m.
- And a libido that sometimes clocked out without notice

Nobody tells you that elevated blood sugar feeds yeast like it's at an all-you-can-eat buffet. Nobody tells you that vaginal health is *directly linked* to your blood sugar levels.

And nobody, I mean nobody, talks about how frustrating and *embarrassing* it can be.

But I'm not here to sugarcoat (pun intended). I'm here to say:

You're not nasty. You're not alone. And you're not broken.

And let me tell you this—when my sugar finally got under control?

Babyyyy, the smoothness came back like a skincare commercial.

I mean, soft. Silky. Not a hint of irritation. I was standing in the mirror like, "Who is she?!"

It was like a whole new lease on my lady parts.

It wasn't just a physical shift—it was emotional too. That smoothness was proof:

My body responds when I care for it. It's trying to heal, not hurt me.

How I Got It Together

Once I understood that the itch wasn't random, I took action. I cut back on sugar-heavy foods (even the sneaky ones like certain fruits and yogurts), took probiotics, switched to cotton underwear, and started actually listening to my glucose meter like it was giving out life advice. Oh—and I went back to my doctor and said, "Look, I need treatment for this yeast situation *and* I need to get my blood sugar in check, or I'm going to scream in lowercase letters for the rest of my life."

Within a couple of weeks of managing my sugar levels better, the itching stopped. Like, *completely*. And that's when I knew: the coochie was never the problem. The sugar was.

Mini Pep Talk:

If you're dealing with the itch, don't suffer in silence. Don't be embarrassed. Don't let anyone tell you it's "just a hygiene thing." You deserve to feel comfortable in your own skin—and your own underwear. Take your power back, one glucose check and one cotton panty at a time.

🎁 Itch-Be-Gone Survival Kit

1. 👙 Cotton undies only, breathable fabrics
2. Unscented, pH-balanced soap
3. 🍲 Probiotics (talk to your doc)
4. Low-sugar diet to control yeast overgrowth
5. 💊 Antifungal cream (yes, keep one ready)

Did You Know?

Vaginal yeast infections can be one of the first signs of Type 2 diabetes—and they tend to come back until blood sugar is under control.

💬 Real Talk Reflection Prompt

How do you handle uncomfortable symptoms that are hard to talk about? What helps you find courage to speak up?

📢 Pull Quote

"The coochie was never the problem. The sugar was."

Bet. Let's keep this train moving—next stop: your eyeballs, which apparently had their own plans. 👀

Chapter 6

Blink Twice if You Can See Me

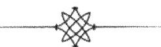

Eyesight going blurry like someone smeared Vaseline on your lenses. One day I was reading a text, and the next, I was squinting like Mr. Magoo. I thought my glasses were dirty. Nope. It was my blood sugar doing optical illusions.

I thought my glasses were dirty. I cleaned them. Still blurry. I squinted so hard I gave myself a headache. That's when I found out diabetes can mess with your eyes faster than you can say "optometrist." It's called **diabetic retinopathy**, and it's one of the leading causes of **blindness in Black adults**. I was walking around half-blind, thinking I just needed new lenses, but what I really needed was to stop playing with my blood sugar. If you've been asking people to read menus out loud, this chapter is for you.

So boom—I'm reading the back of a cereal box one day (don't judge me, it was right in front of me) and I notice I'm squinting like it's written in Morse code. I grab my phone to zoom in and… the screen is blurry too. First thought: "Oh lawd, am I going blind?"

Second thought: "Is it the diabetes?"

Spoiler alert: YES.

Nobody told me diabetes could mess with my vision *before* it messed with anything else. I thought I was going crazy, like maybe I needed glasses or had stared at screens too long. But no, my blood sugar was sky-high, and my eyes were the first ones to snitch.

When Blurry Became My Normal

Before I was diagnosed, I just thought I needed stronger glasses. I'd go to the eye doctor like clockwork—get my annual exam, listen to that little puff of air, get my new prescription, and drop *hundreds* of dollars on new frames. (You know the kind—cute, artsy, "I'm-still-fine-in-a-meeting" glasses.)

Then? A few weeks later—blurry again.

I'd think, *Did they mess up my prescription?*

Buy contacts. Still blurry.

Try to push through—sometimes with double vision, sometimes with a headache, and sometimes just straight up missing people's facial expressions.

One year, I went back to the doctor THREE times.

Every time, they adjusted my prescription. Every time, it still didn't feel right.

It was like my eyesight was in a mood. Like it woke up some days and said,

> "We feel like -3.5 today, actually. And tomorrow? Let's give -6.0. For fun."

Turns out, high blood sugar can make your vision fluctuate like that. It swells the lens in your eye. So when my glucose levels were doing the electric slide, so was my prescription.

I wasn't going crazy.

I wasn't being dramatic.

My vision was literally reacting to what my body couldn't process.

And let me tell you, that realization felt better than any prescription ever could.

How High Sugar = Blurry Vision

Here's the science: when your blood sugar is high, your body pulls fluid from everywhere—including the lenses in your eyes. That messes with your ability to focus. It's like someone put your vision on shuffle. One day you're fine, next day your phone looks like a Monet painting.

This isn't *permanent* damage—yet. But if your sugar stays high, it can lead to **diabetic retinopathy, glaucoma, cataracts**, or even vision loss.

The Frustration Is Real

Let me tell you, nothing tests your patience like trying to thread a needle (or read a text) when your eyeballs are staging a rebellion. I bought reading glasses, squinted through movies, held my phone an inch from my face like a boomer, and still felt like I was walking through life in soft focus.

And then? It would randomly clear up. A few days later, blurry again. That on-again, off-again drama? Classic sign of fluctuating blood sugar.

Especially for Black Folks

Black adults are **2-3 times more likely** to develop diabetes-related blindness than white adults. But we're less likely to get regular eye exams or be told that diabetes is a direct threat to our vision.

And we're often misdiagnosed or dismissed when we say "something just feels off."

How I Got My Sight (and Sanity) Together

- Started checking my sugar every time my vision got blurry. Without fail—*it was high*.

- Went to an optometrist who checked for retinopathy (thankfully, none yet).

- Invested in blue light glasses & screen timers (hello, less eye strain).

- Got serious about my blood sugar numbers. Like *real* serious.

- Added foods that support eye health—greens, berries, omega-3s, and water.

Slowly but surely, my vision stabilized. Not perfect, but I'm no longer living in a fog.

Mini Pep Talk:

If your vision feels off, believe your eyes. They're not lying. Your body is asking for help, not judgment. Don't wait for it to get scary—get it checked early, and don't be afraid to say, "Hey, this doesn't feel right."

🔧 Interactive Elements

✅ Blurry Vision Check-In

1. 📅 When was your last eye exam?
2. 👁 Do your eyes blur after eating?
3. 📉 Is your vision worse when you skip water or meals?
1. Do you need glasses—or new ones?

🎁 Diabetic Vision Care Kit

- Appointment card reminder (schedule it!)
- Blue light filter glasses
- Eye drops for dryness
- Low glycemic snacks to prevent spikes
- Sunglasses (yes, UV matters too!)

💬 Real Talk Reflection Prompt

What would it mean to take your health seriously *before* it gets serious? What's one step you can take today?

Did You Know?

Diabetic retinopathy is the **#1 cause of blindness** in working-age adults—and it can often be caught early with annual exams.

📣 Pull Quote

"I didn't need a new prescription—I needed a new plan."

Chapter 7

Puff, Puff… Nope – The Swelling Nobody Talks About

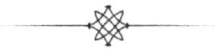

You ever look down and wonder, *"When did my feet turn into memory foam pillows?"*

Like, blink twice and suddenly your ankles are gone, your shoes don't fit, and your body feels like it's holding on to water like it's saving for retirement.

Call it what you want–but it's one of those sneaky symptoms that had me out here googling 'Do diabetics inflate?"

Welcome to the Great Puff-Up.

Also known as: **swelling, edema, bloated Barbie mode, or That Time My Feet Said "We Out."**

💢 What It Actually Felt Like:

Let's talk visuals.

- Feet so swollen I thought I was turning into one of those balloon animals from the county fair.
- Rings wouldn't fit. Socks left imprints. I even had to buy shoes in a size up *temporarily*.
- My legs felt tight and heavy. Sitting down too long? Bad. Standing up too long? Worse.

- Flip-flops? Became my best friends and worst enemies—because baby, *they exposed everything*

My feet were so puffy, I looked like I was auditioning for *Cloudy With a Chance of Foot Pain.*

I'd take off my socks and see stripes from the elastic like I'd been wrapped in deli paper.

Rings? Not happening.

Shoes? Had to size up.

At one point, I swore my legs were humming from the pressure. Like I had built-in subwoofers.

And let's not talk about trying to be cute in heels.

"Girl, why are you walking like that?"

Because, sis… these heels are holding back a tsunami, that's why.

📖 🔍 What's Really Going On:

Swelling is **not** just a cosmetic issue. It's your body's version of a protest sign.

Here's what's actually happening:

- **Poor circulation** (thanks, high blood sugar!) slows blood flow and causes fluid buildup.

- **Kidneys** get overwhelmed → they stop flushing extra fluid efficiently.

- Or you're on **certain meds** (like insulin or blood pressure pills) that mess with fluid balance. Yeah, they like to *hold on* too.

- **High blood sugar** damages blood vessels over time → fluid leaks out where it shouldn't.

Basically, you're part sponge, part science experiment. And if you don't address it, it only gets worse.

☹ Humbling, Humid, and Humorous Moments

- I canceled a whole date because my feet looked like soft serve.
- One student asked if I was hiding snacks in my boots. (I was not.)
- I legit started looking up "fashion-forward compression socks" like I was about to start a blog.

There was a time I tried to force my swollen feet into some pre-diabetes heels. Bad idea.

I got halfway down the hallway and turned right back around.

I was limping like a Marvel villain with a vendetta.

✅ What Actually Helped

Let me save you the trial and error:

- ✨ **Elevate those legs**: Desk, couch, passenger seat—prop them up like they're Beyoncé (yes, even at work. Judge me.)

- ✦ **Compression socks**: (ugly? yes. effective? also yes.).

- ✦ **Watch the sodium**: I had to break up with hot sauce. We're seeing other people.

- ✦ **Drink water**: Sounds backward, but water helps flush excess fluid.

- ✦ **Actually taking my meds right** and following up with my doc instead of playing "Google MD.

- ✦ **Move a little**: Even when you're tired. That circulation needs a nudge.

💬 Real Talk:

Swelling isn't weakness. It's not laziness. It's a loud body trying to whisper that something's off.

And when we ignore it? That whisper becomes a yell—and a hospital visit.

There's no shame in the wide shoe aisle. There's no shame in taking care of you.

You can be cute *and* swollen. But being cute, swollen, and ignoring it?

That's a recipe for regret.

Swelling is your body's way of waving a little red flag. Don't ignore it.

It might not be glamorous—but neither is passing out from fluid overload.

✹ Mini Clapback:

"No, I'm not retaining water because I'm pregnant. I'm retaining water because my pancreas and kidneys are beefing. But thanks for asking." ✓

Chapter 8

When Fine Met Phema

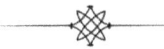

The wildest part of diabetes? I lost weight and thought, *Finally, the jeans fit again.* People were complimenting me. I was feeling snatched. Then the doctor prescribed insulin, and BOOM—weight gain. Insulin is essential, yes, but it also tells your body, "Let's hold onto *everything.*" I went from slim to stuffed in 2 months flat. And for Black women, the pressure to "look good" while managing a chronic illness is *exhausting.* This chapter is about the emotional rollercoaster of losing, gaining, and finding peace in your body again.

The cruel joke: you finally lose weight and feel cute, only to get put on insulin and puff right back up. I was getting compliments: "Wow, you've lost weight!" I was feeling myself. Then came the insulin. Now my jeans are judging me, and my face is rounder than a cinnamon roll (which I *can't* eat, by the way).

I'm not gonna lie—at first, I was *feeling myself.* Pants sliding on easier, face slimmed out, waist snatched. Folks were complimenting me left and right:

> "Girl, have you been working out?" "You look amazing!" "What's your secret?!"

And I'd smile, fake-modest, while screaming internally: *I'M SICK! I'M SICK, Y'ALL!*

The truth was, my body was breaking down, not leveling up. I wasn't losing weight because of discipline—I was losing it because my sugar was sky-high and my body couldn't process any of the food I was eating.

The "Cute" Side of a Medical Crisis

When you have undiagnosed Type 2, weight loss can happen fast. Too fast. Your body can't get energy from glucose (because insulin isn't working), so it starts breaking down fat and muscle instead. That's why I was getting slimmer *and* tired *and* low-key miserable at the same time.

But society loves weight loss. No one asked if I felt okay. They just praised the results like I'd joined a bootcamp and mastered quinoa.

Then Came Insulin… and the Plot Twist

After the diagnosis, my doctor put me on insulin to bring my numbers down. I was scared, but ready to feel better.

What I *wasn't* ready for? The weight gain. My body, now finally processing food correctly, started storing energy again. And baby, it did NOT store it modestly.

The scale crept back up. My jeans betrayed me. And the people who once said "you look so good" now said… nothing. Or worse— "You were doing so well, what happened?"

The Emotional Toll? Real AF.

That glow-up-to-glow-down rollercoaster messes with your mind. I didn't want to be skinny if it meant being sick. But I also didn't want to gain weight from the thing that was *saving my life*. It felt unfair.

I had to relearn what *health* looked like. And more importantly, I had to stop tying my worth to the scale.

Especially for Black Women

We already live in a world that over-polices Black bodies. Add weight gain to that, and suddenly you're lazy, unhealthy, or undisciplined—even when you're literally managing a chronic illness.

We're told to "get snatched" but not told how to *get stable*. That's why this chapter had to be written.

What Helped Me Balance It Out

- Met with a dietitian who understood diabetes and weight cycles
- Focused on *how I felt*, not just how I looked
- Started gentle movement—walking, dancing, stretching—things I enjoy
- Tracked inches and energy instead of pounds
- Gave myself **grace** when my body changed

Mini Pep Talk:

You are not a failure because your body changed. You are not "doing it wrong" if you gain weight on insulin. You are living. Managing. Healing. And that, my friend, is beautiful.

🔧 Interactive Elements

✅ Body Reality Check-In

- ✨ Am I treating my body with kindness—or criticism?

- 💼 Have I been tracking only my weight, or also energy and mood?

- 💬 Have I spoken to a professional about safe, balanced weight goals?

🎁 Feel-Good Toolkit (Beyond the Scale)

- Journal for energy & mood tracking
- Non-scale victories list (pants fit, slept well, better focus)
- Favorite comfy outfit for "blah" days
- Mantras like: *"Progress, not perfection"* or *"My body is not the enemy"*

💬 Real Talk Reflection Prompt

How do you define health for yourself—not society, not the 'gram—*you*?

Did You Know?

Insulin is a hormone that promotes fat storage. Weight gain on insulin isn't failure—it's biology.

📢 Pull Quote

"I looked better sick, but I feel better now. I'll take *feeling better* every time."

📖 Real-Life Sidebar: The Ozempic Reality

Let's have a moment of realness. I walked into my doctor's office frustrated and bloated.

"Everybody else is using diabetic meds to get *snatched*," I said, "and here I am *gaining* weight like it's a competitive sport. Can I get *something* out of this diagnosis?"

I looked my doctor dead in the eye and said, "Listen. The world is losing weight on diabetic meds. I gained twenty pounds in two months. Give me whatever they're giving the skinny girls, because this ain't it."

That's when the conversation about **Ozempic** started. I didn't jump on the hype train to drop dress sizes—I got on because I was genuinely trying to manage my blood sugar. But still, I was hoping I'd at least get a little *something* out of this Type 2 madness.

Spoiler alert: It worked a little—but not like social media promised. Because when you're *actually* diabetic, the rules hit different.

This part of the journey? Full of surprises. And more than a few side-eyes.

🌸 Shareable Moment:

Create a quote or meme that empowers you in your sugar journey:

"I'm sweet enough without the sugar.

#TheHoneyBunRedemption"

Chapter 8 (Deeper Cut)

The Weight Drop That Made Me Cute Then Insulin Said "Psych" – ft. Ozempic Lies & Real-Life Results

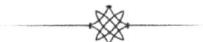

Let's talk about **Ozempic.**

The world is out here treating it like a miracle juice. Celebs on red carpets whispering about it. Instagram influencers swearing by it. "This diabetic shot changed my life!" they say.

And meanwhile, I—an actual diabetic—was prescribed Ozempic and sat there like, "...So where's *my* skinny?"

When the "Wonder Drug" Does Nothing But Stabilize

Here's the kicker: everyone else was losing weight off this stuff like it was a cheat code. But me? Nada. Not a pound. And trust—I waited. Took it faithfully. Did the diet. Watched my portions. Checked my sugar like a hawk.

And yet... my jeans still fit the same. The number on the scale didn't budge. The only thing that got slimmer was my patience.

But hey—my blood sugar stabilized. My A1C went down. My pancreas? She's clapping in the background.

So yes, it "worked."

But in a world that glamorizes thinness, when you *don't* get the side effect everyone else is bragging about, it feels like another punch in the gut.

The Truth About Ozempic (and Others Like It)

Drugs like Ozempic (semaglutide), Wegovy, Mounjaro—they're all part of this new class of GLP-1 receptor agonists. And yes, they're effective. They *can* reduce appetite and delay stomach emptying, which can lead to weight loss.

BUT here's the truth they don't put in the TikToks:

- If your insulin resistance is severe, weight loss might not happen right away—or at all.
- If your body's been running on empty (aka undiagnosed for a while), it's going to prioritize *stability* over slimness.
- And if you're truly diabetic, your body's response is **not** the same as a normo using the med recreationally.

So yeah—I got my blood sugar down. I felt better. But I also felt… *forgotten.*

Emotional Whiplash, Part 2

Nobody claps for you when your sugar is stable. There's no applause for normal A1C levels. No compliments for not passing out today.

But lose 20 pounds on a shot you don't even need? Suddenly you're "inspiring."

That's the problem. The praise is *misplaced.*

What I Had to Remember

- I'm not here to be a weight loss success story—I'm here to *survive*.
- My value isn't tied to whether or not I dropped dress sizes.
- Stabilizing your sugar? That's the real glow-up. That's the invisible win.

I still take Ozempic. Not for the 'gram. Not for a bikini. But because it helps keep me here. And I've decided *that's enough*.

🔧 Interactive Elements (Expanded)

📕 Medication Reality Check Journal

1. 💉 Medication I'm currently on:
2. 📈 What improvements have I *actually* seen?
3. 🤢 What side effects do I *hate*?
4. What is this doing for my *health*, not just my weight?

📣 Mantras for When You Feel Invisible

- "My progress is not measured in pounds."
- "I am not a side effect. I am a whole person."
- "Stability is success."

💬 Reflection Prompt

How do you handle disappointment when the "magic fix" doesn't work for you? What's something that *is* working for you right now—even if it's not glamorous?

Did You Know?

Studies show GLP-1 medications are **less likely to cause dramatic weight loss** in people with long-standing Type 2 diabetes, especially when insulin is also involved.

📣 Pull Quote

"Ozempic didn't make me skinny. It made me *stable*. And honestly? That's what I needed more."

Chapter 9

Double Trouble – When Diabetes Brings Along High Blood Pressure

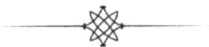

Listen. If diabetes is the loud, messy cousin at the cookout, high blood pressure is the one who sits in the corner real quiet—until *bam*, he flips the table.

I thought I was dealing with *one* chronic illness. ONE. I barely had time to wrap my head around glucose numbers when here comes my doctor, talking about:

> "Your blood pressure is up too."

Ma'am?? Sir?? How much do you think I can handle in a week?!

Diabetes and Hypertension: The Toxic Tag Team

Turns out, having diabetes **doubles your risk** of developing high blood pressure. Why? Because both conditions are about how your body handles fuel, pressure, and inflammation. When your blood sugar is high over time, it damages your blood vessels. Damaged vessels = higher pressure = double trouble for your heart, kidneys, and eyes.

This isn't just an "add-on." High blood pressure makes diabetes complications way worse. And guess what? You don't even feel it most of the time.

Silent but Deadly

That's the scariest part. High blood pressure doesn't always give you signs. No dizzy spell. No headache. No nothing. You just wake up one day and your doctor is giving you "the look" after they check your numbers:

> "Are you stressed?" "Have you been watching your salt?" "You exercising?"

Meanwhile, I'm like: "Sir, I'm watching my carbs, my sugar, my insulin, my weight, and my sanity. You want me to watch *salt* too?!"

Black Women and the Hypertension Hustle

Let's get real: Black women are **80% more likely** to develop high blood pressure than white women. And we're more likely to have it *younger*, more *severely*, and with *more consequences*.

Why?

- Genetics
- Stress (yes, racism counts)
- Socioeconomic barriers
- Lack of access to affordable, culturally competent care
- AND being constantly told to "lose weight" instead of treated like human beings with complex needs

My Reality Check

I was already tired from managing diabetes. Adding hypertension made me want to give up. Another pill. Another tracker. Another number to worry about.

But I had to flip the script and see it for what it was: a *warning*, not a death sentence.

What Helped Me Reclaim Control

- Got a **home blood pressure monitor** so I could track on my own terms
- Reduced processed salt (bye Lawry's, hello Mrs. Dash)
- Moved more—even just dancing in the kitchen counts
- Started taking my BP meds *consistently* (not just when I felt "off")
- Prioritized **mental health**—meditation, therapy, boundaries, and naps

Mini Pep Talk

Managing diabetes is hard enough—but if high blood pressure shows up, don't ignore it. This is your body waving a red flag. Take the warning seriously, but don't let it scare you into silence. You have tools. You have options. And you don't have to be perfect—just *present*.

🔧 Interactive Elements

✅ Blood Pressure + Blood Sugar Log

Create a 7-day tracker to jot down:

- Blood sugar (AM/PM)
- Blood pressure (AM/PM)
- What you ate
- Movement that day
- Mood/stress level

(You'd be surprised how much that stress column connects with your numbers!)

🎁 Hypertension Survival Kit

- BP cuff for home
- Salt-free seasoning blends
- Chill playlist or meditation app
- Journal for venting the stress *before* it hits your pressure
- List of small movement ideas (stretching, walking, dancing, marching in place)

💬 Real Talk Reflection Prompt

What's one small change I can make this week to support both my heart *and* my sugar?

📣 Pull Quote

"I didn't ask for diabetes and hypertension to be roommates. But now that they're here? I'm running the house."

Let's pivot with flavor, because oooooh... nothing cuts deeper than watching someone bite into hot, buttery or lemon peppery wings when you're sitting there with a plate of sadness and grilled chicken. It's time for the real talk:

Chapter 10

The Wingstop Breakup

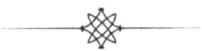

Listen. I've been through breakups. I've let go of toxic friends. But giving up food?

That was a heartbreak I did *not* see coming.

No one prepares you for the grief that hits when your go-to comfort foods become enemies. When the snacks that raised you—chips, cakes, cornbread, fried everything—start to feel like betrayal on a plate.

But it's real.

The cravings.

The nostalgia.

The frustration.

The mourning.

A Love Story with a Sad Ending

Now let me tell you about one of my most *painful* goodbyes…

Wingstop.

More specifically—those sweet, salty, crispy, tangy **Lemon Pepper wings**. Baby, those wings held me down through breakups, bad days, celebrations, and casual Tuesdays. That flavor? That crackly skin? That greasy little paper bag that made your car smell like heaven?

I was in *love*.

But when diabetes entered the chat, my body said:

"You can't do this anymore, sis. He's not good for you."

And just like that, I had to break up with Wingstop. Cold turkey. I mean, I was deleting the app, driving past the location like it was my ex's house, rolling up the window when I smelled that lemony fried goodness in the air.

I was heartbroken.

Later though, when I got more in control—when I learned how to manage my sugars, plan ahead, balance my meals—I went back.

Not for the relationship.

Just for the *casual date*.

I'd treat myself, just not cheat myself. Two wings, maybe three. Paired with water, veggies, and intention.

That was the glow-up: not never eating my favorites again, but learning how to flirt with them responsibly.

Food Was More Than Fuel—It Was Family, Culture, and Comfort

For me, food was **ritual**.

- Sunday dinners that started Saturday night.
- Mac and cheese that could win awards.

- Pound cake so good it made you want to call your ex and apologize.

So when diabetes said "Nope!" to half the things I grew up on? I felt robbed.

I missed the *experience* of eating—of not having to read every label, calculate every carb, or ask "Will this spike my sugar?"

It's Okay to Grieve the Old Plate

Yes, it sounds dramatic. But it's valid.

You're not just changing what you eat—you're changing the way you *relate* to food.

That's loss. And it's okay to be sad about it.

But here's the flip side...

You Can Still Find Joy in Food (Seriously)

I had to stop thinking in terms of "What can't I have?"

And start asking, "What *can* I have that still feels like me?"

Because food isn't the enemy.

Blood sugar chaos is.

I learned to:

- Recreate my faves with swaps (hello almond flour cornbread!)
- Experiment in the kitchen like a mad scientist

- Season EVERYTHING—don't you dare bring me bland health food
- Let myself *enjoy* food again, guilt-free and sugar-stable

Yes, I Still Cheat. No, I Don't Feel Bad.

Every now and then, I eat the bread. I eat the cake. And guess what?

I plan for it.

I test.

I correct.

And I *move on*.

Because this isn't a punishment.

It's a *practice*.

Interactive Elements

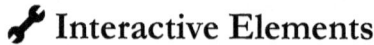 Craving Tracker

Keep it real:

- What am I craving?
- When do I crave it?
- What's really going on? (Stressed, bored, emotional?)
- What healthier option might actually satisfy me?

🍽 Reclaim Your Joy Recipe List

Start a running list of:

- Meals that keep your sugar steady AND bring you joy
- Healthy versions of comfort foods that actually hit
- New flavors/spices you've fallen in love with

Example:

✓ Air-fried chicken with Cajun spice

✓ Cauliflower mac with sharp cheddar

✓ Sugar-free peach cobbler (don't knock it 'til you try it)

📖 Food Journal Prompt

"The dish I miss most is _____ because it reminds me of _____. I want to honor that memory by finding a version that works for my health *and* my heart."

📣 Pull Quote

"I don't miss the food—I miss the freedom. But now, I'm finding freedom in feeling good after I eat."

Ooooh yes! Welcome to the **Breakup Menu**—where we lay our food relationships bare and walk through the drama like it's a telenovela. You didn't just change your diet... *you went through something.*

🍽 The Breakup Menu: From Toxic Love to Healthy-ish Healing

🍽 The Food Fling	💔 Breakup Status	😩 Emotional Stage	💅 Glow-Up Replacement
Wingstop Lemon Pepper	Ghosted, deleted, re-followed	Denial Bargaining Balance →	Homemade air-fried lemon pepper wings
Mac & Cheese	Long-distance relationship	Grief & Betrayal	Cauli-mac with sharp cheddar and spice
White Rice	"We need space"	Acceptance	Brown rice, cauliflower rice, quinoa
Sweet Tea	Filed for a sugary divorce	Anger	Stevia-sweetened tea with lemon
Honey Buns	Restraining order issued	Depression	Sugar-free cinnamon mug cake (trust me!)
French Fries	Toxic, and we both knew it	Relapse Recovery →	Baked sweet potato wedges or turnip fries
Pancakes & Syrup	"It's not you, it's my A1C"	Regret	Almond flour pancakes with sugar-free syrup

| Soda (Coke, Pepsi) | Blocked & reported | Empowerment | Sparkling water with a splash of lime |

💔 Healing Notes:

- **You can still "see" them… just don't move back in.**

- Balance is key: You can visit your faves occasionally *without moving back to your old zip code.*

- Be kind to yourself. You're not failing—you're evolving.

📖 Journal Prompt:

"Which food was hardest to let go of, and what memory is tied to it? What new version of that dish would feel like a celebration *and* self-care?"

📣 Pull Quote:

"You can love a food and still leave it behind. Especially if it no longer loves you back."

Chapter 11

Pills, Prayers and Process of Elimination

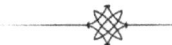

Let's talk about the *real* part of managing Type 2 diabetes: trying every combination of medication, food, schedule, and mindset like you're solving a Rubik's cube... *blindfolded*... while it's on fire.

This chapter is about the trial-and-error phase—and let's be honest, it's *mostly* error before you find your groove.

The Medication Maze

The pharmacy was giving me options like I was ordering off a chaotic fast food menu:

- Metformin
- Ozempic
- Jardiance
- Insulin (basal or bolus? short-acting or long-acting?)
- Glipizide
- Januvia

I wanted to scream: *Can I just get the combo that doesn't make me bloated, tired, moody, or have to pee every 20 minutes?!*

Spoiler: It doesn't exist. But over time, I found what worked *for me*.

Here's how I figured it out:

- **Kept a log** (yes, even when I didn't feel like it)
- Noted when my sugar was high *and* how I felt—headaches, fatigue, weird cravings
- Took notes to my doctor like I was building a case file: "Exhibit A: This dose makes me dizzy by 4 PM."

Eventually, we created a combo that didn't leave me feeling like a zombie. Progress.

Food Is Not the Enemy... But Also Not My Bestie

Look. You will *hear* a lot about "diabetic-friendly" foods. Most of it? Boring, dry, and depressing.

Early on I was living on egg whites, air, and hope. But I couldn't live like that long term.

So I had to redefine my plate:

- Learned about *pairing* carbs with protein
- Switched to **slow carbs** (brown rice, sweet potatoes, whole grains)
- Found swaps that didn't feel like punishment (zucchini noodles? not today, Satan. But cauliflower mash? Not bad.)
- Discovered seasoning is your friend—spice makes anything feel like soul food

Exercise... but Make It Make Sense

People kept telling me: You just need to move more!

And I was like, "Move where? Move how? I'm tired!"

But here's what clicked: it doesn't have to be the gym. It just has to be movement.

My favorite diabetic workouts:

- Dancing in the living room (Beyoncé is cardio)
- Walk-and-talk phone calls
- Grocery store laps (before I buy the snacks)
- Marching in place during TV shows

15 minutes here, 10 minutes there—*it counts*.

Mental Health: The Secret Weapon

Nobody talks about how exhausting diabetes is mentally. The guilt. The shame. The "I should've caught this sooner." The "What did I eat?" panic spirals.

I started journaling. Then meditating. Then therapy.

And baby, that helped *more* than some of the meds.

Taking care of my *mind* helped me make better choices for my body. Because when you believe you're worth saving? You fight harder.

Real Wins That Aren't On a Chart

- Fewer sugar crashes
- Waking up with energy
- Not crying at the pharmacy
- Understanding labels

- Feeling in control—even when I slip up

🔧 Interactive Elements

What's Working Worksheet

- Medications I'm on:
- Side effects I notice:
- What's working well:
- What's NOT working:
- Questions for my next appointment:.

🍽 My Real-Life Food Wins

- Healthy swaps I actually like:
- Go-to meals that don't spike my sugar:
- Snacks that satisfy cravings:

📈 My Progress Tracker (Beyond the Numbers)

- Today I:

1. Drank enough water ✅
2. Moved my body ✅
3. Took my meds ✅
4. Gave myself grace ✅

Mental Health Check-In

On a scale from "I got this" to "I'm losing it"—how am I really feeling today?

📣 Pull Quote

"Treatment isn't one-size-fits-all. It's trial, error, and triumph. One adjustment at a time."

Yesss, let's dive all the way in. This next one? It's for every person who's been judged, questioned, or dismissed because they "don't look sick." Buckle up:

Chapter 12

"I Don't Look Sick" – Fighting a Disease That People Can't See

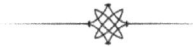

You ever had someone look you dead in the face and say,

"You don't *look* like you have diabetes"?

Like there's a diabetic *uniform*. Like I'm supposed to be falling over with a glucose monitor glued to my forehead, foaming at the mouth in aisle 3 of Target.

Nah, baby. This disease? It's silent. It's slick. And it'll tear you up on the inside while you smile, laugh, and carry on like everything's fine.

✧ I Don't Look Sick — But I Am.

There's this thing that happens when you live with a chronic illness and still know how to smile.

People assume you're fine.

You're glowing? Must be healthy.

You showed up? Must be good.

You cracked a joke? Can't possibly be struggling.

But let me tell you about this one tournament. I was there, in my role, doing what I do—supporting students, showing up with professionalism and warmth, and giving energy I didn't even have.

But behind the scenes? I was spiraling.

My blood sugar was dropping. I hadn't had a real break, let alone a meal.

I quietly asked to be rescheduled so I could eat. Politely. Kindly. Gently.

I even smiled.

They said, *"You look fine."*

And scheduled me for another round.

They couldn't see the migraine blooming behind my eyes like a thunderstorm.

They didn't know my hands were shaking from hunger and stress.

Because I didn't *look* sick. Because I didn't scream. Because I didn't collapse.

Because I smiled.

Afterward, I retreated into myself. Shut down. People asked,

"What's wrong with her?"

"Why she got an attitude?"

"She was just smiling earlier…"

Yes. I was. But behind that smile was a woman trying to regulate her blood sugar while also regulating her emotions in a space that made no room for either.

That's what people don't understand about invisible illness.

It's not always tubes and crutches and visible pain.

Sometimes it's smiling through a migraine.

It's judging a debate round with shaky hands.

It's advocating for yourself quietly—because you're tired of explaining—and being ignored anyway.

The Problem With Invisible Illness

Here's the thing: when you don't look sick, people don't take you seriously.

- Your fatigue gets brushed off as laziness.
- Your mood swings? Oh, you're just being dramatic.
- That foggy brain, the headaches, the chronic thirst? "Maybe you need more sleep."

No, ma'am. No, sir. I have a whole-body condition that's messing with everything from my nerves to my emotions. But because I'm not in a hospital bed or visibly wasting away, folks assume I'm exaggerating.

The Internal Battle Is Real

Some days I can function just fine. Some days I feel like a superhero. And some days? I can't think straight, my body aches, and I'm riding the blood sugar rollercoaster wondering if I'll make it to 3 PM.

But I still show up. For work. For family. For everybody.

That doesn't mean I'm not struggling. It just means I've mastered the art of "looking okay."

When Even Doctors Don't Believe You

Whew. This one hurts. I've walked into appointments describing real symptoms, only to be met with:

> "Well your numbers aren't *that* bad…"

> OR

> "Maybe you're just stressed."

Gaslight, gatekeep, glucose.

The worst part? As a **Black woman**, I'm more likely to be dismissed, downplayed, or misdiagnosed. Studies have shown that Black women's pain, fatigue, and symptoms are often ignored or underestimated.

So we get quiet. We stop asking questions. We stop advocating.

Reclaiming My Voice

I had to learn to be *louder* than my symptoms.

- I started writing things down before appointments.
- I asked for second opinions.
- I switched providers when they didn't listen.

- I gave myself permission to *not be okay*—even if I looked fine.

To the Outside World: Stop Judging Our Journey

You don't know what it takes to manage this every day. You don't see the fear behind every bite. You don't know the panic of waking up dizzy, shaky, or not at all. You don't live in this body—*I do*.

So stop telling me how healthy I look. Ask me how I *feel*.

🔧 Interactive Elements

🎭 Invisible Symptom Tracker

Use this weekly log to capture what others *can't* see:

1. Physical fatigue: 😒 😐 😁
2. Mood swings: 😱 🙂 ☺
3. Brain fog: ☁ 🚫 📋
4. Joint pain: 😕 🙂 💪
5. Blood sugar highs/lows: ⬆☐ ⬇☐

📋 Speak Up Script

Use this at your next appointment:

> "I understand my numbers may not look extreme today, but I'm experiencing [symptom]. I'd like to discuss options to manage it better, because it's affecting my daily life."

Reflection Prompt

When was the last time I didn't feel believed? How did I respond—and how do I *wish* I had responded?

📢 Pull Quote

"Just because I don't look sick doesn't mean I'm not fighting for my life every single day."

Ohhh yes—we're riding this wave all the way in now. Time to get deep deep. Let's talk about that guilt, that shame, and that annoying voice in your head that says, "You should've known better."

Chapter 13

Diabetic Guilt, Shame, and the "Should've Known Better" Spiral

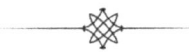

The moment the doctor said *"Type 2 diabetes,"* I heard nothing else. Just that heavy, echoing guilt bomb go off in my chest.

I sat there thinking:

"How did I let this happen?" "I knew better. I saw the signs." "I failed myself."

Nobody warned me that a medical diagnosis could feel like a moral failure.

The Shame Game Is Real

As soon as people find out you're diabetic, the questions start coming like pop quizzes:

- "So what did you eat to get it?"
- "Is it because you're overweight?"
- "It runs in your family, right?"
- "You know you have to cut out sugar now, right?"

There's this **blame culture** around diabetes that doesn't exist with other illnesses. Like you brought it on yourself. Like you didn't pray hard enough, walk far enough, or turn down enough biscuits.

But here's what no one tells you:

You can eat perfectly, exercise daily, and *still* end up with diabetes. Genetics. Hormones. Stress. Chronic inflammation. Life.

It's not just about food. It's never been *just* about food.

The Lies I Told Myself

I carried that guilt like it was a badge of honor:

- "I deserve this because I didn't take better care of myself."
- "I should've gone to the doctor sooner."
- "I can't talk to anyone about it—they'll judge me."

But here's the truth: beating myself up didn't help my sugar. It just made me too ashamed to ask for help.

Unlearning the Shame

Healing started when I stopped asking:

"What's wrong with me?"

And started asking:

"What do I need right now?"

Because guilt drains your energy.

Shame keeps you silent.

But *grace?* Grace gives you room to breathe—and grow.

You Are Not a Failure. You Are a Fighter.

You showed up to the appointment. You got the diagnosis. You made a plan. You took the meds. You asked the questions. You're reading this book right now.

That's not failure. That's *power*.

🔧 Interactive Elements

📓 Guilt Dump Journal Prompt

Write it out. No filter. No judgment. Just raw truth:

"I feel guilty about _____."

"I've blamed myself for _____."

"What I needed back then was _____."

"What I deserve now is _____."

Tear it out. Burn it. Keep it. Whatever you need to release it.

🧠 Mindset Shift Check-In

"If my best friend had diabetes, would I speak to them the way I speak to myself?"

If the answer is no? It's time to be kinder to *you*.

🌱 Affirmations for the Comeback

- I am not my diagnosis.
- I am learning and growing every day.

- I forgive myself for what I didn't know then.
- I deserve care, support, and healing.
- I am doing my best—and that is enough.

📣 Pull Quote

"Guilt didn't save me. Grace did."

Chapter 14

Sex, Skin & Sugar – The Intimate Side of Diabetes

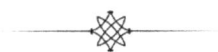

Let's not play cute.

Diabetes doesn't just show up in your bloodwork and your grocery cart—it shows up in your **bedroom**, your **bathroom mirror**, and the **way you feel about yourself** when nobody's looking.

And yet... nobody *warns you* about *this* part.

So let's talk about it.

☹ Let's Start With "Down There"

Itching. Burning. Dryness. Discomfort.

And not in a sexy, Fifty Shades of Grey kind of way.

Sometimes it felt like my body was mad at me. I was doing "all the things"—taking my meds, drinking my water—and still dealing with:

1. Yeast infections on repeat like a toxic ex
2. That unbearable itchy feeling that makes you want to rub yourself raw
3. White discharge that had me Googling everything at 3 a.m.
4. And a libido that sometimes clocked out without notice

Nobody tells you that elevated blood sugar feeds yeast like it's at an all-you-can-eat buffet.

Nobody tells you that vaginal health is *directly linked* to your blood sugar levels.

And nobody, I mean nobody, talks about how frustrating and *embarrassing* it can be.

But I'm not here to sugarcoat (pun intended). I'm here to say:

You're not nasty. You're not alone. And you're not broken.

And let me tell you what happens when your sugar is finally under control.

Baby, it's like a spa day down there.

That skin? Smooth. Soft. Calm.

No itching. No irritation. No weirdness. Just peace. I remember touching my skin one day—just casually—and thinking, *"Oh, okay silky! I see you!"*

Babyyyy, the smoothness came back like a skincare commercial.

I mean, soft. Silky. Not a hint of irritation. I was standing in the mirror like, "Who is she?!"

It was like a whole new lease on my lady parts.

It wasn't just a physical shift—it was emotional too. That smoothness was proof:

My body responds when I care for it. It's trying to heal, not hurt me.

After all that time suffering in silence, I finally felt like my body was working *with* me instead of against me.

That moment deserves a whole standing ovation and a scented candle.

💔 When Your Body Doesn't Feel Like Yours Anymore

Let's talk about skin.

Dry. Ashy. Cracked.

I used to lotion up like I was prepping for a Soul Train line. But with diabetes? Sometimes I felt like I was moisturizing a **desert**.

- Elbows like chalkboards.
- Shins that looked like they'd been dusted with flour.
- Skin so dry it *hurt* to move.

Then came the **dark patches**, the discoloration, the weird rashes.

You start avoiding mirrors.

You start hiding parts of yourself.

You start forgetting that you are STILL worthy of feeling beautiful, desired, and whole.

💋 The Bedroom Blues

Let's be real: when your sugars are high, your desire is *low*.

Your body is tired. Your mind is foggy. And sometimes you'd rather nap than be touched.

I've been there.

And when your partner doesn't understand—or worse, takes it *personally*—it adds another layer of guilt to an already heavy load.

But here's what I learned:

- Honest conversations change everything.
- Intimacy doesn't disappear—it just shifts.
- When you start to feel *good* again physically, the desire often returns too.

So be patient with yourself.

And remind your partner: this body is doing the most. Show it some grace—and some love.

✨ But Here's the Flip Side…

When your sugar is controlled, your skin glows.

Your energy rises.

Your desire comes back swinging.

You see yourself again. You feel your *fine* again.

There's no better sexy than *feeling good in your body* again. And that? That's the part worth fighting for.

🔧 Interactive Elements

📧 Journal Prompt: Body Realness Check-In

"What's one part of my body I've judged harshly since my diagnosis? What's one way I can care for or celebrate that part with love instead?"

🛁 Self-Care Checklist for That Skin & Sugar Life

- Fragrance-free, hydrating lotion (use daily)
- Cotton underwear (breathability is key!)
- Unscented soap for intimate areas
- Keep blood sugar in check (less sugar = less yeast)
- Sexy playlist for when you're feeling yourself again

☐ A Few Bedroom Truths

- It's okay to pause.
- It's okay to say "not tonight."
- It's okay to say "YES, tonight!"
- It's okay to explore new ways of pleasure that feel *right* for you now.

📣 Pull Quote:

"Diabetes may shift your body, but it doesn't steal your beauty, your worth, or your right to pleasure."

Yessss. Let's go there. Because diabetes doesn't stop for date night, and explaining your blood sugar to someone mid-cuddle is not in the romance movies.

Chapter 15

Love, Lust, and the Low Sugar Text – Dating & Relationships with Diabetes

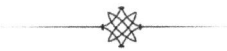

Let's be honest.

Diabetes is *already* a full-time relationship—with your body, your meds, your blood sugar monitor, and your carb count.

So throwing another human into the mix? Whew.

This chapter is for anyone who's ever wondered:

- "When do I tell them I have diabetes?"
- "Will they judge me when I pull out my meter at dinner?"
- "Can I still feel sexy with an insulin pump on?"
- "How do I explain needing a snack after sex without sounding like I'm dying?"

💬 The First Date Disclosure

There's no *right* time.

Some folks drop the "D-word" over appetizers. Others wait until date #3.

Either way, it's not a confession—it's a fact. You're not asking for permission. You're setting the table.

Sample Script (aka The Chill Drop):

"Just a heads up, I have Type 2 diabetes. So if you see me checking my blood sugar or whipping out snacks like it's Halloween, that's why."

If they flinch or say something dumb? Cool. You just saved time.

🔪 The Bedroom Breakdown: Sexy Time & Sugar

Listen. There's nothing sexy about cramping from low blood sugar mid-stroke.

But also—there's nothing unsexy about **taking care of your body**.

Here's what comes up and how to handle it:

1. "Do I leave my pump on?"

Girl, it's up to you. Some people rock their devices with pride. Others disconnect or tuck it away.

If they're the right person, they're gonna be focused on *you*, not your Dexcom.

2. Low Blood Sugar After Sex is Real AF

The energy. The sweating. The blood flow. Your body's like, "Was that cardio? Cool. Let's crash."

Have a snack nearby. Tell your partner what to look for. And don't be afraid to say,

"Hold on, I need to check my sugar real quick."

That's not unsexy. That's being alive to go another round.

☺ When They Don't Get It

You will date people who mean well but don't get it.

- "Can you just cheat on your diet this once?"
- "You look healthy to me."
- "You just need to drink more tea."

And you might feel tempted to shrink yourself. To minimize. To laugh it off.

Don't.

You deserve love that learns. That listens. That Googles. That asks,

"How can I support you better?"

💘 When They Do Get It

Oh. My. God.

When someone:

- Packs snacks for you
- Notices when you're "off"
- Asks about your doctor's visit
- Doesn't flinch when you inject insulin

- Holds you while you wait for your sugar to rise again that's intimacy. That's the soft, safe love you *deserve*.

💬 Journal Prompt:

"What do I want my next partner (or current one) to understand about my diabetes experience?"

📣 Pull Quote:

"If they can't handle your glucose monitor, they don't deserve your glow-up."

Let's gooo! Pivoting right into the **Survival Kit chapter**—*because dealing with diabetes means you're basically a medical MacGyver: always ready, always equipped, and maybe carrying a glucose tab in your bra (hey, no judgment).*

Chapter 16

The Diabetes Survival Kit – What's in Your Bag, Sis?

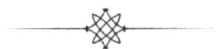

Living with diabetes is like running a 24/7 body-monitoring business—no PTO, no breaks, no HR department.

So if you're gonna survive (and thrive), you need a **kit**. Not just the physical one in your purse or car, but the emotional, mental, and lifestyle one too.

Let's break it down.

🎒 The Real-Life, In-Your-Bag Kit

The Basics:

- Glucose meter + test strips
- Lancets (because yes, we're still pricking fingers like it's 2005)
- Alcohol wipes
- Emergency snacks (peanut butter crackers, glucose tabs, fruit snacks—stash *something*)
- A small water bottle (because you are never not thirsty)

💊 The Backup Plan:

- Extra meds or insulin (if you're using it)

- A pen needle or insulin syringe
- Medical ID bracelet or wallet card
- Copy of your prescription, just in case life gets dramatic

⚡ The "Oops" Items:

- Hand sanitizer (because you've tested your sugar in some wild places)
- Lotion (for that ashy skin situation)
- Panty liners or spare undies (hello, unexpected leaks from all that peeing)
- Small mirror (to check your eyes, mouth, or mood without facing a whole mirror meltdown)

The Mental Survival Kit

Diabetes is more than physical. It messes with your *mind*, too.

▮♀ Emotional Essentials:

- A journal or notes app to brain dump on bad days
- A playlist that hypes you up (or calms you down)
- One person you can text: "I'm struggling today" without explaining everything
- Sticky notes of encouragement: "You're doing your best." "You got through yesterday, you'll get through today."

✨ Affirmations to Repeat:

"I am not my numbers."

"I'm allowed to rest."

"I am adapting, and that is brave."

"I still get to live fully and joyfully."

💻 The Digital Kit

These are the apps, websites, and hacks that keep you organized and sane:

- **MySugr / Glucose Buddy / Dexcom apps**: for tracking
- **Health reminders** on your phone: meds, water, blood sugar checks
- **Instacart**: because grocery store runs when you're low on energy are *not it*
- **Spotify**: because music is medicine too
- **A "Diabetes Notes" folder**: log symptoms, doc questions, weird moments to ask about

🎒 The "Just In Case" Self-Compassion Pack

Because some days will suck. And on those days, you'll need to remember:

- You are not lazy. You are managing an invisible full-time job.
- Your worth is not tied to a number on a meter.
- You don't have to explain your choices to anyone.

- You are allowed to cry. To cancel plans. To eat the cookie. To say no. To say yes.

- You are allowed to start over as many times as you need to.

📖 Journal Prompt:

"What do I need in my life kit—not just my purse—to feel prepared, grounded, and safe as I manage diabetes?"

📣 Pull Quote:

"My survival kit isn't just full of tools—it's full of grace."

Yessss—let's talk about the real, raw, ridiculously relatable breakdown. Because every diabetic knows: no two days are the same. One minute you're good, the next you're cussing out your meter and threatening to eat a cinnamon roll just to prove a point.

Chapter 17

The 7 Types of Diabetic Days – A Humorous Breakdown

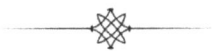

Because if you don't laugh about it… you'll cry in the pharmacy parking lot with low blood sugar and a bag of glucose tabs you don't even like.

☯ 1. The "I'm Basically a Doctor" Day

You wake up. Your blood sugar is in range.

You eat something responsible and leafy.

You walk 10,000 steps before noon.

You log everything in your app.

You drink so much water you basically live in the bathroom.

You're like, *"Should I host a TED Talk? Am I the blueprint?"*

Warning: This day usually precedes…

💥 2. The "WTF Is Happening" Day

You did everything the *same* as yesterday.

Same food. Same meds.

And yet—your sugar is sky-high like it's trying to reach Beyoncé.

You sit there like:

"So the math's not mathing? The insulin is insulin-ing, but the sugar is sugarin' harder?"

Cue rage-eating a boiled egg out of spite.

💀 3. The "Did I Die and Come Back?" Day (aka The Low)

You feel weird. Sweaty. Dizzy.

Then you check your sugar and it's like... 47. ☐☐

You grab the nearest sugar like it's a life raft.

Half a juice box. A piece of candy. That expired granola bar in your car. You'd eat a cough drop if it had carbs.

Once you're stable again, you look around like:

"What just happened and why do I feel like I just came back from the afterlife?"

4. The Zombie Day

Blood sugar's normal, but you? You're *tired tired*.

You slept 8 hours but woke up feeling like you worked a double shift in your dreams.

You drag yourself through the day. You forget your keys. You forget your name.

You question everything.

"Am I tired from diabetes, or is this just adulthood? Or both? Either way, I need a nap and a snack."

5. The "I Don't Care, I'm Eating It" Day

You've been good all week.

Then someone walks by with a honey bun, and you remember who you used to be.

You don't count carbs.

You don't log anything.

You don't care.

You eat the thing.

And you *savor it*.

"I'm not reckless. I'm just rebellious with seasoning."

(And don't forget: it's not about never having treats—it's about planning. But sometimes… forget the plan.)

6. The Mindful Queen Day

You drink your herbal tea.

You meditate.

You eat slow.

You wear loose, flowy clothes and call it "honoring your pancreas."

You check your sugar and say things like "I receive this number."

You post an IG story that says *"Diabetes doesn't define me."*

It lasts 24 hours, just like your resolve.

7. The "Cold, Clinical, Just Get Through It" Day

No emotion. No drama.

You test. You inject. You log. You sip water.

It's not good, it's not bad—it's just business.

Your face says: "I am the CEO of Glucose."

Your heart says: "I'm tired."

But you do it anyway. Because that's what surviving looks like sometimes.

📣 Pull Quote:

"Every diabetic day has a vibe. Some are divine, some are demonic, and some are just—*meh*. But you keep showing up."

🎯 Interactive Element:

📅 ☐ Which Diabetic Day Are You Today?

Doctor Mode

WTF Mode

Just Came Back From the Dead

Sleepy Zombie

I'm Eating It, Leave Me Alone

Mindful Queen

Cold & Clinical

Rate your day. Own it. Then keep pushing.

Final Chapter

Still Sweet – A Message from Me to You

So here we are.

If you've made it this far, you've laughed, maybe cried, definitely scratched something that was probably diabetes-related, and most importantly—you *stayed*. You stayed with yourself. Through the weird symptoms. The scary diagnosis. The food temptations. The "why me" moments. The slow victories.

Let me say this plainly:

You are not broken. You are not to blame. You are not a burden.

You are someone navigating a condition in a world that barely talks about it—and you're doing it with grit, grace, and maybe a little bit of lemon pepper seasoning.

Type 2 diabetes doesn't define you. But it *does* invite you to show up. For your body. For your peace. For your future self, who still deserves joy, softness, and that fly outfit you've been saving for "when I feel better."

✹ Call to Action: Don't Just Read—Respond

This isn't just a book. It's a call to **do one small thing**.

Not everything. Not perfectly. Just one thing.

- Book that follow-up appointment.
- Replace *one* snack with something that loves you back.

- Text your group chat and say, "Y'all—I'm managing my sugar now. Hold me accountable."

- Or maybe just drink some damn water. (Seriously. Hydrate.)

Whatever you do, do it with the knowing that **you're worth the effort**. You deserve to feel good in your skin, in your body, in your life.

📢 Final Word:

"The diagnosis may have shocked me. The honey bun may have tried to take me out. But I'm still here. And now, I'm choosing me—every messy, powerful, healing day."

Now go. Live. Love. Laugh.

And read your nutrition labels.

— With love,

✨ Still Sweet. Still Standing.

Okay, I lied! One more final word!

This book was never just about diabetes.

It was about reclaiming power, telling the truth, laughing through the mess, and saying:

"I'm still here. And I'm not going out over a honey bun."

💬 **If nothing else, remember this:**

- You are not alone.

- You are not your numbers.

- You are worthy of softness and strength at the same time.

✅ Before You Go: Your Final Checklist

I've forgiven my past self.

I'm loving this current version of me.

I'm not doing this perfectly, but I'm doing it.

I have a plan—or at least a water bottle and a snack.

I'm still funny. Still fine. Still fighting.

📲 Stay Connected

This journey doesn't end here.

Come find me. Share your story. Let's keep this conversation—and this community—alive.

Facebook: @RaiRenea

Instagram: @rairenea

Email: renea.moss@reneasworld.com

Hashtag: #StillSweetBook #honeybunredemption

Tag me when you're walking into that doctor's appointment, skipping past the snacks, or just feeling yourself in the mirror. I wanna celebrate you.

♥ With Heart, Humor & Healing,

www.ingramcontent.com/pod-product-compliance
Lightning Source LLC
Chambersburg PA
CBHW072056290426
44110CB00014B/1710